Alpha Male

The Path To
Hardcore Natural Bodybuilding

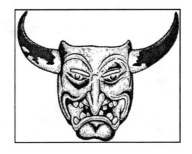

Go Heavy or Go Home

Sam DeLucia
First Edition 2001

COPYRIGHT

Published by William Delucia, 6250 Telegraph Rd. # 2106 Ventura, CA 93003. Email: psycholifter@psycholifter.com

©2001 Sam Delucia. All rights reserved. No part of this publication may be reproduced, stored in a retrieval system, or transmitted in any form or by any means, electronic, mechanical, recording or otherwise, without the prior written permission of the author.

ISBN# 0-9709601-0-7

Attention(Disclaimer): Always consult a Physician before undertaking an exercise program or diet.

Dedication
Dedicated to my Valkyie Dawn. My buddy Gidion.

Thanks
Artist Jerry Beck and Iron Asylum. Strength Coach Kirk Adams. Classic Bodybuilder Ed Corney. Editor in Chief Adam Barlow (Why do you have to do two reps more than me?).Cabel. Jerry Wilhelm. Rob. Bill Delucia. Joe Pasko. Steve Reeves. Lou Ferrigno. Arnold Schwarzenegger. AC/DC. Thor. Dorogard.

The Inventor of the Bench Press.

CONTENTS

1   **ONE** *Initiation into the Brotherhood*
- Quiz: Are You Ready to Become Hardcore?

8   **TWO** *The Unobtainable Goal*
- Magazines
- Supplements
  - Truth on Protein Supplements
  - Truth on Creatine
  - Truth on HMB
  - Truth on DHEA
  - Truth on Androstenedione
  - The Only Real Supplement You Need Is…

Psycho Insert/ The Brotherhood in Motion

15   **THREE** *Become the Alpha Male*
- Alpha Male
- Pride of Being Natural
- Sacrifice
- Limits
- Visualization/Imagery
- Progress

21   **FOUR** *Psycho Trainer Guide*
- Psycho Trainer Method of Inspiration?
- Signs of a Good Set
- "I'm Ready, What Can I Do to Become a Psycho Partner?"
- Beware the Slacker, in All His Shapes and Forms.
- The Everyday Lifting Rut, and the Lying Principle
- Motivation During the Set is Important

- Pay Attention. Demand More.
- Push Yourself....The Boastful Claim Method.

Psycho Insert/ Barbarian Slave

31 FIVE *Build Mass with Massive Lifts*
- Intro
- Getting Ripped vs. Putting on Mass
- Exercises
    - Biceps
    - Triceps
    - Trapezius
    - Shoulders
    - Chest
    - Abs
    - Back
    - Forearms
    - Quads/Hamstrings
    - Calf
- Free Weights vs. Machines
- Sets, Reps, Intervals
- Intensity
- How Heavy is Heavy?
- The Program
- Basic Workout
- If You Plateau On One to Two Exercises For Basic Workout
- If You Plateau On Three or More Exercises for Basic Workout
- Plateau Buster
- Plateau (Advanced Techniques)

53 SIX *Eat Meat: The Real Guide to Nutrition*
- The 40-30-30 Training Diet

- Helpful Facts and Hints
- Truth on Water
- Truth on Carbohydrates
- Truth on Protein
- Recipes

62 SEVEN *So You Want to Compete?*
- Part I – The Journey Begins
- Part II – The Time is Near, The Eve before De struction

74 EIGHT *Hardcore at Home and on the Road*
- Home Gym
- Basic Needs
- Optional, but if you can get one
- The Other Essentials
- How To Save Money
- Commercial Gym

79 NINE *Cream of the Crop: The Best Natural Bodybuilding Sites on the Internet*
Psycho Insert: Prophet of Progress

83 TEN *Best Emails*

88 ELEVEN *Best Mantras to Keep the Blood Pumping*

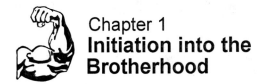

Chapter 1
Initiation into the Brotherhood

I know who you are. You've been lifting for a year or so, chasing the ultimate bodybuilding physique. You've seen the ads in the magazines: "Bigger Biceps in Four Weeks!" or "Workouts for Killer Quads!" You want 22-inch biceps and a 54-inch chest, all this *plus* six-percent bodyfat. You've taken all the right supplements, followed the latest pro routines, and went to the gym faithfully, hell bent on getting huge.

But something's wrong. You've made admirable gains but have hit a wall. Your arms are bigger but not huge. Your quads are larger but not freaky. Veins the size of a radiator hoses don't travel down your arm. You're starting to notice other things also. How about the time you ran out of protein powder for a month and still made gains without the chocolate shake. You went on vacation another time and didn't go to the gym for two weeks. When you came back you were a little stronger. You think, "Hey, that's strange."

Another time, exhausted from overtraining, you were up into the wee hours of the night channel surfing and stumbled across a "Natural Bodybuilding Contest" on ESPN. The contestants were ripped and had nice size but they weren't the gigantic monsters you're used to seeing in the muscle mags. "Why are they so much smaller than the professional bodybuilders?" you ask yourself. You start thinking about your other friend at the gym who has trained for five years and is about the same size as one of these natural guys - and he's been training for awhile now. Hmmm...

This makes you think, "Am I the only one who sees this?". The answer is no, you are one of many. You're just now starting to see the light but just can't grasp it yet. You're ripe for the truth now.

Here's the simple truth of it all: if you lived to be five hundred years old and went to the gym everyday, you will never be some freaky mound of flesh. No magic routines, no supplements, no special techniques are going to make you as large as the professional bodybuilder. Why is that? Because you are natural and they are not....plain and simple. Then why won't the magazines say those the bodybuilders aren't natural? *Money*. Why won't the bodybuilders say they take growth hormone or anabolic steroids? *Money*. The bodybuilding corporate machine has to keep you coming back for more and more. The supplement industry is a five billion a dollar year industry and someone has to buy them.

With the power of the growing Internet, a new world of discussion groups, websites, and online e-zines has emerged. People just like you, fed up with the commercialism of weight training and bodybuilding. People want truth, not truth connected to a program at the bargain price of $29.95 or a new supplement. That's exactly how I felt when I created my website the Brotherhood *(www.geocities.com/getoffmeyou)*. I was tired of all the useless information. I wanted a site for lifters who were natural; a site that contained real information. I wanted a site for those who had focus and were driven to succeed naturally. I was overwhelmed by the response.

Yes, there are many all over the world just like you. I received emails from frustrated lifters on every continent and over thirty different countries. These lifters didn't want commercialism; they wanted reality. They took their training seriously. They trained hardcore and thought hardcore. They just never had a voice before...but that's before the Internet came. There are many of us out there. We're a tight group. A brotherhood of weight trainers and bodybuilders who think pure is good and training hardcore is better.

Pumping iron to these guys transcended exercise and just wanting to "look good". Those are tangible goals for all us, even among our brotherhood. We all want to gain mass. But, somehow pumping iron becomes more than mere exercise. It's a way of life. Even if you layoff for a month or even a year, you still hear the "Call". You always come back. You feel guilty as hell when you miss a workout. People think you're crazy. Seem familiar?

Hardcore and natural is a way of life. It's in your heart as well as the mind. We believe in hitting the body hard with the basics. Lift heavy, use the basic heavy movements, eat, sleep, and give your body time to recuperate. That's the secret. It's not a magic supplement, it's not the new workout in the muscle rags, and it's not a quick fix. You're not going to go out and put on thirty pounds of muscle in three months! It takes persistence, commitment, will power, and the vision. You have to be the rock in the gym that's there day after day, month after month, year after year.

Gaggles of newbies always seem to rush into the gym after Christmas to lose twenty pounds for summer. They come to socialize, using a high volume, five-day a week workout consisting of a plethora of isolation movements. Yes, you've seen them. "Pretenders," that's what the Hardcore call them. They'll use the workout *du juor* from a fitness magazine. They end up burning out in a few months and are subsequently gone from the gym. They ignore the basics. Instead of building a brick house of a body and then defining it later, they perform sets and sets of lightweight isolation movements and wonder why they haven't grown bigger muscles. Of course, the remedy must be supplements and a new workout. That's how it starts - a vicious cycle for the uninformed that never ends. Here's the secret, folks: lift heavy, eat right, sleep, and *stick with it!* For god's sake, stop changing workouts! It's not hard. It's just most people don't have the guts for intense sessions over a long period. They want results today and aren't willing to work and wait for tomorrow for what they want.

My advice is stay the course and enjoy your training sessions. With lifting comes camaraderie with your friends, the feeling of success as your bicep grows another half-inch or the confidence you gain as you hit a new personal record. Overall, the enjoyment of pumping iron comes from within. It's the clank of the weights, the gritty hard driving music, and the natural high of intense lifting. It's the pump you receive from the satisfaction of a good workout. It doesn't matter where you lift, home gym or regular gym, the love of iron is with you wherever you go. As walls or barriers are thrown in your path, you don't step aside. You move forward because you know in your heart, "Here comes the wrecking ball!"

Are You Ready to Become Hardcore?

Take this quiz (Answer yes or no):

1. Is any training that's not intense and heavy as hell an embarrassment for you to perform?
2. Wouldn't be caught dead in the gym in lycra bicycle pants? Do you see others that do as a long lost member of the Village People?
3. See sickness as an annoyance that holds up training?
4. Would jump on the tailgate of a bus just to get to the gym?
5. See supplement ads the same as ads for adding new hair or ads for penile implants?
6. Put Muscle and Fitness magazine on the floor for the dog?
7. Sees blood as extra sweat?
8. Sees Suzanne Summer's AB Cruncher® as a great nacho server?
9. Wonder why guys in the muscle mags are always greased up like an overstuffed pigs?
10. Want to lynch whoever has Mariah Carey blasting over the stereo in the gym?
11. Want to see Weider puke after you put him through a real man's workout?
12. Would eat bark off a tree just to get some protein?
13. Does the idea of a hole in the wall gym with hard driving rock 'n roll and a horde of iron plates causes instant drooling?

If your answer to the vast majority is yes, then proceed. It's time to hear the truth and get some unfiltered information. As the character Morpheus said in the movie *The Matrix* to Keanu Reeves's character, Neo, "Hold out your hands. In my right hand is a red pill and in my left a blue one. You take the blue pill and the story ends. You wake in your bed and you believe whatever you want to believe. You take the red pill and you stay in Wonderland and I show you how deep the rabbit-hole goes. Remember that all I am offering is the truth. Nothing more."

Which pill do you choose?

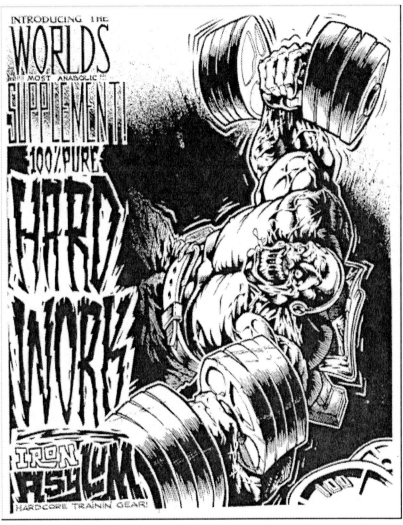

Courtesy of **Iron Asylum**. Visit **www.ironasylum.net** for more awesome designs!

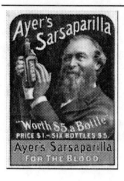

Chapter 2
The Unobtainable Goal

Supplements – Modern Snake Oil

What if you got this offer in the mail?

Listen up! How would you like to own a piece of a multi-million dollar industry? Well, you too can be a Professional Bodybuilding Mogul. Here's what you get:

> ➤ A magazine that offers inane workouts and worthless advice. A publication full of model bodybuilders who built their muscles on anabolic steroids (but your reader doesn't need to know that); and, in fact, your reader will think it all came from supplements and that's exactly what you want them to think!

> ➤ A supplement product line in a 5 billion dollars a year worldwide market - the readers of your magazine will buy gobs of the stuff hoping to obtain the physique of one of their favorite chemically enhanced bodybuilders. Put whatever you want in the bottle, the FDA won't check!

> ➤ Hold bodybuilding contests for chemically enhanced bodybuilders who are on your payroll. Disregard any

aggressive drug screening for illegal steroids, it's bad for business!

> Just sit back and let the money roll in!
> **Call Now! Only $19.95!**
> **1-800-RIP-OFFF**

Sounds good, doesn't it? The object of *Hardcore Natural Bodybuilding* is to see professional bodybuilding for what it really is and set you down the path to real muscle growth. What you see above is the real state-of-affairs in the professional bodybuilding world of today. It all starts with the magazines.

Magazines

The magazines are the main tools used by the professional bodybuilding industry to reach their main audience. The muscle rag offers articles on diet, gossip, and of course the new end-all-be-all workout that will send you to huge biceps heaven. Included inside is the ever present surplus of pictures of greased up bodybuilders grimacing through some imagined workout, or layouts of models in skimpy clothes laying provocatively over any imaginable piece of gym equipment. All this to sell you supplements which is their main aim. That's where the real money is. In a 5 billion dollar a year industry, if you can get just a piece of it, it could mean *millions*!

Magazine	Supplement They're Pushing
Muscle and Fitness	Weider
Flex	Weider
Muscle Media 2000	EAS
Muscular Development	Twinlab
Ironman	Muscle-Link

Supplements

If the magazine is the golden goose then the supplements are the golden eggs. Readers seem to think that if they follow the workouts and take the right supplements they're going to be the next big thing. Not true. Check out this fact:

> In 1994, the FDA no longer tested supplements and relaxed its requirements of the supplement manufacturers. The manufacturers can make claims as long as they have research to back it up, usually done by labs they pay. If the manufacturers state or give untrue claims for the supplement, they get a letter of reprimand. If it happens again, a referral is made to the Justice Department. So overall, the burden of policing the industry is left to the manufacturers. "I could fill capsules with sugar and sell them as a new miracle supplement," says Anderson, PhD., "Unless someone dies from them, I could market them with no problem." Scary, huh?

Here are some facts on some popular types of supplements:

Truth on Protein Supplements

"But I have yet to see a strength-training athlete who's already not eating enough protein." says nutritionist Susan M. Kleiner, Ph.D., R.D., co-author of Power Eating. "They're already focusing on it, having an extra chicken breast here, a glass of skim milk there. That's fine…..There's no advantage to taking protein as a supplement. It's not absorbed better. It's not utilized better." In fact, extra protein may put undue stress on your kidneys over time.

Truth on Creatine

Unless you're lifting weights constantly or playing a sport that requires sudden bursts of speed, then creatine is no help. Studies have shown a 2-6 pound gain over a four to six week period but the studies cannot determine how much of the gain is just plain water weight. All creatine is not equal. Advance Supplement Testing Systems checked 107 supplements to see if the chemicals matched the claims of the labels and found that 53 were off by more than 20%. Kirk Adams, Strength and Conditioning Coach, adds, "The 'real deal' is still to be determined. There have been studies that have shown positive, negative, and inconclusive findings. The long-term safety of creatine is unclear. Again, creatine should be thrown in with all other supplements. There are simpler, safer, and less expensive ways to make gains in your training."

Truth on HMB

The claim of HMB is it can prevent the breakdown of protein in your muscle tissue. It works in animals but this claim has not been proven to work on humans. The University of Memphis did a study on HMB and found that there were only modest gains at best.

Truth on DHEA

DHEA is converted by the body into testosterone. Kreider, at University of Memphis, says that there are no studies that have proven that this conversion spills over to any muscle gains for those that lift weights.

Truth on Androstenedione

Researchers at Iowa State University studied 20 men during an eight-week training program. Half of the group was given a placebo while the others were given a 300mg dose of Andro. After the study was over, the researchers could not detect any strength difference between the two groups.

Says Kirk Adams, Penn State Strength and Conditioning Coach about supplements, "Supplements are just that-- supplements to doing the right thing which includes training hard, eating properly and getting plenty of rest. If any of those three are missing, there is no reason why anyone should consider taking supplements. For the most part, supplements are over priced and their benefits are greatly exaggerated. Beyond that, we do not know the long-term safety of most of the supplements out there. First, your genetics determine most of your physical abilities and development, or lack there of. From there, hard work, proper nutrition and rest can take you a long way. There were plenty of strong individuals before there were high priced supplements. There is no 'easy way' or 'magic formula.'

Supplements are needed if you're gonna get big. Wrong. Mankind has been packing on muscle mass since the beginning of time. Do you think people have only been muscle-bound since 1970? The blacksmith was the biggest man in his village because he worked with heavy metal all day not because he ate whey protein and used creatine. Everything you need is in nature whether it's for energy or muscle repair. Supplements should be used to supplement your diet; they shouldn't be your diet. Supplements can be helpful but you don't need them - if you're convinced you do you're brainwashed.

The Only Real Supplement You Need Is...

Hardcore Natural Bodybuilding is about total *natural* bodybuilding. Hardcore lifting, sweat, dedication, and that's all. Professional bodybuilding is a farce. The contests aren't really about who has the best body, but who balances their drug cycling with their training the best to become the biggest freak of nature. If you think professional bodybuilders get their body from diet, training, and lots of sleep, then you better WAKE UP! If you believe what the muscle mags are feeding you, then you'll probably believe that in next year's Mr. Milky Way Galaxy contest, Santa Claus is gonna edge out the Easter Bunny for best chest. The *real* hardcore lift with no other help than a jug of water, rippin' tunes, protein, and helluva lot of attitude.

Interview With 1970's Star Bodybuilder Ed Corney
Ques: How do you feel about young people looking to guys in the mags as heroes - thinking if they take supplements and use their workouts, they're gonna be big just like them?
Answer: Good luck. Those guys take steroids to gain an edge. As long as there is a market for that body-style they'll continue.

Rock On.

The Brotherhood in Motion

By Kindredkind (Yahoo Club)

Enters the gym the mind in a Zone
Has no yuppie friends and works out alone
Raggedy sweat shirt and weightlifting gloves
Walks toward the iron, pain is what he loves
Admirers and passers watch, and he pays no mind
For they are weak, and not of his kind
Sinew burns from the weight and from the pain
What he wants is gain, and the spirit doesn't wane
Others cringe, from pain he endures
Living the life of iron is the only cure
He cries to the Brotherhood, the last rep, last set
Unable to complete it, was his only regret
Bleeding sweat, bone through the flesh, he's bar none
Anguish, cramps, veins popping, his workout is done
He crawls from the gym, for the workout was good

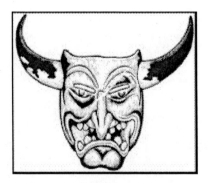

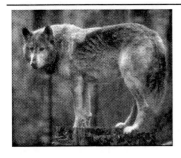

Chapter 3
Become the Alpha Male

"There is no way to underestimate the importance of the mental aspect of lifting. During your lift, you need to be completely focused on the task at hand and breaking through the limits set by your last workout. Personally and professionally, I've seen what a positive, intense attitude can accomplish."
   - **Kirk Adams, Strength and Conditioning Coach.**

Alpha Male

In the animal kingdom, often the dominant male in the group is known as the *Alpha Male*. He is the leader, protector, and warrior; the top dog. In a wolf pack, the Alpha Male wolf is a force to be reckoned with. In those terms, I think it is important to see yourself as the Alpha when it comes to weight training. There must be no backing down as you test the limits of your strength. You are the Alpha when you are in the gym. You must have confidence, maybe even a little fear too. Fear can elevate adrenaline levels. When you get on that bench under a load that you never have lifted before, see yourself as the Alpha. You are on the road to actualize your true potential and no one is going to get in your way to your goal. You are the Alpha, the top dog, a determined unstoppable force.

The human race is one of the most powerful species to walk the planet. There's a reason humans reign supreme in the natural world. For example, in the ages of yore when we humans were uncivilized, we were predators, hunters, and animals. We are capable of explosive power and great feats. Tap into that power - we all have it even though it is buried deep.

Go to the gym focused. Don't worry about any outside distractions. This is your time, a mission to realize your full potential. When I'm in the gym, I'm the one sweating profusely wearing an old T-shirt, ratty high tops, and whatever shorts were clean (or not). I'm unlike the other trainers walking around with lat syndrome (that is, walking around with their arms away from their bodies for no apparent reason, as if they have *huge* lats) in too tight tank tops, cut off sweatshirts, and $100 sneakers talking about how much they can bench. I'm there to work and keep myself focused.

Pride of Being Natural

In my mind, I see being totally natural as a badge of honor. I even take it a step further by not using supplements. All my nutrition comes from what I can buy in the grocery store. It's the attitude of separating yourself from the masses. As you read in chapter two, most supplements are crap anyway. You don't need them, but the bodybuilding industry says you do in order to meet your goals. How untrue. They have a financial investment in you believing in that fallacy. They may reap in millions but they're not going to get my dollar.

Steroids are the same. Anyone who sticks needles or takes pills to gain muscle is taking a great health risk and is *not* considered natural. It takes hard work and dedication to be a Hardcore Natural.

Being natural is just that, being natural. Take the pride in the way the iron feels in your hands, the effort you put forth, and the rewards you reap from your trials in the gym. Good diet, heavy training, and plenty of rest is all you need. If you look at statues of athletes from ancient Greece or Rome, you can see the muscle mass that the ancients could put on. They didn't stick needles in their rear. They didn't take L-Glutamine. There's a pride in being natural, a pride in being connected to something that separates your training from the masses.

Sacrifice

Often fitness experts say you must find some free time in the day so you can workout. It must be convenient. Well, today's life is busy and you're never going to have time. To fulfill your potential takes dedication and sacrifice. The following quotes from Vince Lombardi, ex-Super Bowl Coach for the Green Bay Packers, demonstrate the willingness to sacrifice to be Hardcore.

- "If you quit now, during these workouts, you'll quit in the middle of the season in a game. Once you learn to quit it becomes a habit. We don't want anyone here who'll quit."

- "Fatigue makes a coward of us all. When you're tired you rationalize. You make excuses in your mind. You say, 'I'm too tired, I'm bushed, I can't do this, I'll loaf.' Then you're a coward"

> Defining the willingness to suffer: "It means you got home a little later, a little wearier, a little hungrier, and with a few more aches and pains."

Limits

You have no limits. Get that into your head right now. Your limits are self-imposed. You have yet to realize your full potential so you really don't know what your limits are. When you change the way you train, you change your limits. Even if you plateau in your lifts there are ways to bust a plateau. If you continue to make progress, then you have yet to hit your limit. Open your mind to what is possible. Let your body tell you what is possible and leave your mind out of it. If your max in the bench press is 250 pounds, that is your max at this moment in time. The future is yet to be determined.

Arnold Schwarzenegger in his book, *Encyclopedia of Bodybuilding*, used the following example:

Before 1970, people believed that lifting 500 lbs. was impossible. In 1970 it was finally achieved during the Olympics. Then in the next few months after, 500 lbs. was lifted many more times by others. Why? Mental barriers. Once one person did it, others believed they could do it too. The mind is very powerful, focus and believe in yourself and you *will* be successful.

Visualization/Imagery

Visualization is an important component in harnessing your own power during intense training. When the training becomes more intense over time, you must be able to quiet your mind and visualize yourself succeeding in your lift.

Imagine that you are on your fourth set on squats, your heaviest set. You did five reps last week and are shooting for six reps this week. You must then focus intensely on your lift. First, you quiet your mind by blocking out the distractions around you including talking to your lifting partner. In that moment of silence, focus on the lift before you. Think about all the things that need to be done correctly for the squat. See yourself getting under the bar, shouldering the weight, and backing away from the rack. Visualize yourself during the lift going to the floor, keeping your back straight, and exploding upward for your goal, the sixth rep. Do this a few times, but most important visualize yourself succeeding. Does this guarantee success? No. What it does guarantee is that you are on the path to giving it all you have to give.

Imagery is different than visualization. Using imagery you imagine an event or something that motivates you to higher levels of intensity. For example, imagine directing all your stress of that guy who cut you off on the road into that barbell before you. Imagine yourself an ancient warrior training for his next battle. Feel the bloodlust. Anything it takes to drive your mind to focus all energy into the task before you.

When I'm in the gym, I often lift alone. In between sets, I pace back and forth keeping my mind focused on the next lift. I visualize the lift and succeeding in it. My headphones are usually pumping in some heavy metal riff driving my mind forward. It's the only way can I keep myself on track.

Progress

As you go through your training life, redefine what progress means to you.

Do Not's:

- ➢ **Do Not** compare yourself to bodybuilders in magazines - it's unrealistic.
- ➢ **Do Not** compare yourself to others as a way to measure your gains - compare yourself to yourself.
- ➢ **Do Not** compare yourself to supplement ads - you're not going to pack on 30 pounds of muscle in 60 days.

Progress can mean many things, whether it's getting to the gym everyday, putting on five pounds of muscle, adding ten pounds to your max lift, or achieving an 1/8th inch growth on any given muscle. It's all progress.

Redefine what progress means to you. Develop your goals, keep a journal and record progress. Feel great when you accomplish your goals, or fuel your determination to move forward if have yet to meet the goal.

Your future is in your own hands.

Chapter 4
Psycho Trainer Guide

"Psycho Trainer Guide" By Joe Pasko
(http://www.scri.fsu.edu/~pasko/psycho.html)

This website is one of my favorites and nothing shows you more than this guy what it's like to be Hardcore Natural. So here is an excerpt of the Psycho Trainer:

The PSYCHO Trainer Method of getting HUGE.

Copyright 1995 Joe Pasko... No part may be copied or reproduced without written consent.

DISCLAIMER... You could get HURT/INJURED and or HUGE when applying the training methods described below. THESE TRAINING METHODS DESCRIBED BELOW ARE INTENDED FOR INTERMEDIATE TO ADVANCED LIFTERS...

So you want to get BIG and get big FAST ?? If you're like most guys, you've been working out a few times a week and are seeing some decent results, but this isn't enough. That workout rut has taken hold, and results are coming more slowly. What you need is a kick in the complacency. Summer is here, and looking like a slug just won't do. I'm going to introduce a workout philosophy here that has worked wonders with a number of rut stuck couch-potato turned muscle-men. I call it the Psycho Trainer method of inspiration.

Psycho Trainer Method of Inspiration?

Yes, there are two parts to the Psycho Trainer method of getting HUGE quickly:
1. A sadistic partner.
2. Some sadistic exercise methods.

Make no mistake about it, this workout is going to hurt, and it will hurt a lot (you'll learn later that this is a good thing.) There are a few general benchmarks to the workouts that will let you know if you're doing them correctly.

Signs of a Good Set:

It really sucks and hurts (this is a general guideline, below we'll outline what constitutes proper hurt and suck).

- You can't move that well the next day after doing an exercise.
- You can't move that well two days after doing an exercise.
- During an exercise you hear weird animal noises, then realize your making them.
- Your face changes more than 4 shades of red, purple, or black during a set.
- You see stars, get tunnel vision, and then come-to with a bar resting comfortably on your neck.

"Sounds great, but how do I do it?"

I'm glad you asked. The first thing you'll need is a good workout partner or two (two is better than one, as it reduces the possibility of one person wimping out and dragging the intensity of the workout down to a sane level.) Whether the partner is stronger or weaker than you is irrelevant, attitude is everything (the more sadistic, the better.) The next step is to become a psycho partner yourself. This will allow you to push your partner hard, thus making him/her push back harder. Revenge is a great motivator for these types of workouts.

"I'm Ready, What Can I Do to Become a Psycho Partner?"

To truly become psycho, we need to study one of the most psychotic individuals of our current day and age and emulate him. Rent the video Full Metal Jacket, and pay close attention to the drill sergeant. This sergeant is probably the best role model for the psycho trainer. He elevated recruits to physical levels that they didn't think they could reach, all through fear, intimidation, force of will, and humiliation. This is a good thing.

Beware the Slacker, in All His Shapes and Forms.

The arch nemesis of the psycho partner is the slacker. You need to find when and where your partner is slacking, and this may not be obvious. If your partner lifts 185 lbs. on bench for 10 reps without a spot, this is a sign that he needs more weight (sometimes he'll even grunt a bit to make you think that he's working, don't be fooled). This is the "It's heavy, I'm going to stay at this weight next set" variety of slacker. Don't let your partner get away with this. If you can do 10 reps of something without a serious spot, it's time to increase the weight. INSIST that the partner up the weight and go for a few less reps, (in this case, say 205 lbs. for 6 reps). Many people have unconsciously put self-imposed limits on what they can lift. Don't buy into these limits, force your partner to smash these barriers.

The next variety of slacker is the "I'm just going for reps this set" kind. Ok, using light weight and going for reps can be a good thing, but now let's really go for some reps, not just 10 or oooohhh 12 reps, let's get psycho. Twenty reps should be the minimum for this person, 30 or higher is better. If they can do 12 reps without a spotter, they can do 20 with a psycho spotter. Again refer to the above signs of a good workout to judge whether your partner is putting out an earnest effort.

The Everyday Lifting Rut, and the Lying Principle:

Lying to your partner is one of the best ways to snap them out of the usual rut. Universal machines are the best for this type of inspiration. If you're doing an exercise, say cable rows, and your partner sits down and tells you to put the pin in at 150 (he usually does 10 reps, but insists that it's heavy), have some fun. Put the pin in 170, and use some of the motivational methods listed below to force him to squeeze out at least 8, then berate him for not getting 10. If your partner tries to avoid this by setting his own pin, don't worry, this can be overcome in a few ways. The best is to point out a nice looking female, and as the would-be-slacker looks, drop the pin down a few plates....Cha Ching. If you simply can't fool, shame, or trick your partner into doing more weight, INSIST that he get at least 12 reps.

Motivation During the Set is Important

Total effort should be given to each and every set after a warm-up. There is no excuse for just doing a few reps and putting the weight down. Below are some of the better phrases that are good to scream at your partner during lifts. Anger, fear, and humiliation are the cornerstones of the motivation.

- Was effort expensive today, you couldn't get much?
- Lift you worthless piece of S--t.
- I don't mean to say anything, but my girlfriend lifts more.
- You lift like old people F--k, slow and ugly.
- Of course it's heavy, that's why they call it weight.
- That's not bad....for a girl.
- I've seen your pool cleaner lift more......hey wasn't he at your house today with your wife while you were at work ?
- Worthless must have been on sale, it appears you stocked up...
- That's OK, just take it easy this set, By the way, how was that McDonalds you had for lunch today?

Feel free to improvise on the above list. Screaming at your partner with a fervored intensity is important. Sell the concept that he's worthless unless producing total effort every set (laughter works well here also). Again, see Full Metal Jacket for details. The louder you scream, the better. Public humiliation can be extremely motivational. Try to anger your partner (make sure that he's already lifting, lest you become the focus of the anger rather than the weights.)

If your partner can talk during a set, or right after it, they were not lifting with psycho levels of effort and concentration.

Up the weight, force more reps, and use motivational phrases to increase the mental and physical focus of the workout.

Pay Attention. Demand More.

If you see that your partner is dying, and only has 1 rep left, scream to get at least 3 more and spot him (Spot slowly, and don't give too much help. The lifter should be purple by the time the third rep hits the top.) Know your partner, and know his limits, push him beyond those limits, and insist that he do the same. Again, use the above effectiveness gauge to judge if they proper effort is being put forth. Demand total effort, be uncompromising.

Push Yourself....The Boastful Claim Method.

If you are stronger than your partner, never fear, you too can apply the psycho methods to achieve great results. Exercises where reps are important are a great candidate for the Boastful Claim Method. If you know that your partner can do about 6 pull-ups, offer to do as many as he does TIMES TWO. This will motivate him to do more, just to hurt you, and motivate you do more, to save face. These are both good things. If you have two partners, both weaker, it's ok, modify the boast to "As many as all of you plus 1". Never let the weaker partners get the best of you in these contests. Make it a matter of pride and a challenge to your manhood. Stupid testosterone games are great for this type of training. If you are the weaker partner, jeer at the stronger if he fails to double you in reps or live up to a boast. Continue to rub his nose in it for at least the remainder of the workout.

If you are the roughly the same strength as your partner, let it rip. Pull'em out and see who's bigger on every set. Make it a competition. Be PSYCHO. Bet beer, money, and bragging rights on exercises. Laugh at the loser of the competition, don't be the loser. If you are the loser, beat him on the next exercise. Crushing total effort should be the goal of every set. Only this level of intensity will bring the quick and extreme results that you desire.

Barbarian Slave

by tolkein_1999 (Yahoo Club)

Your feet go down the steps into the cave gingerly. Your movements pensive. You can feel the heat from the fires from below. You think of what brought you to this moment. First, it was the avoidance of the magical formulas almost force-fed to you from the other guards. Huge freaks of nature with abnormal muscles. Guards, slave masters. All part of the empire of evil Josev Veider. Veider promised all the slaves that they would be strong as his guards. Hollow promises and propaganda. You didn't believe, most did. Almost all of the workers who wanted to be strong paid Veider for his magic formulas and never attained their goals. You knew better. Your father had told you to make yourself strong. You had to become like the iron itself. The iron was strong, unyielding. It heard not the rantings of Veider but only its own sweet call from the forge fires, heavy hammers, and sweat of determination. That is how you become a weapon of iron, your father said, become iron yourself.

You enter the bottom of the cave and look around its confines. There are others here. Others that noticed your denial of the magic formulas. The training of your body through exercises taught to you by your father. Long you trained with the heaviest objects you could find. Sometimes long into the night when others had long been asleep.

The others said nothing. Their faces said everything. They were strong too. Muscles made of sweat, blood, and iron. This was your test for the Brotherhood. A group of rebellious barbarian slaves. A slave just like you. You look to the center of the room where a stone dais long and narrow was placed. You know the test, the one your father took long ago.

As you lay down on the dais, the drums and low chanting begins. A secret ceremony of the Brotherhood. Your heart starts to race but you calm yourself purposely. You try to focus on the test in front of you.

Four elders bring to you Barbellk, the ancient black iron weight of ages forged in the eternal fires of Grathis. Barbellk was a long rod almost as long as a man was tall. On each end was a massive Iron Ball forged in the form of a screaming skull. It was said the weight was tremendous, that men had been crushed under its weight only to die in obscurity and failure. The guards of Veider feared the artifact.

Barbellk was placed on your chest by the elders and you grabbed the black iron shaft on each side of your chest. It was all you could to keep the weight from crushing you. Just as the chanting and the drums were reaching a crescendo, the cacophony stopped. The only sound that filled the room now was that of the crackling fires and your trancelike breathing. You focused your mind and put forth all the knowledge given to you by your father. With all your god given might you pushed up the crushing weight to a position a few feet above you. There you stopped. The test was over, you had passed. The others and the elders cried in praise. The elders moved forward to grab the weight. But surprising to all including yourself, you let the weight drop down once again to your chest. The room was dead quiet. With Herculean effort you pushed the obelisk up a second time.

As the elders took Barbellk from you, you looked around the room. They saluted you, pounding a fist their chest. You were accepted. You part of the Brotherhood. A Weapon of Iron. A Solider of Iron. Veider's days were numbered.

If this doesn't psyche you up, what will?

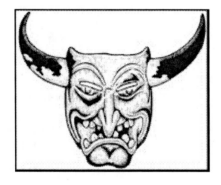

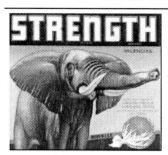

Chapter 5
Build Mass with Massive Lifts

Intro

If you were to look in any month's issue of any popular bodybuilding rag, there would undoubtedly be some big print on the cover with titles like "Build Massive Biceps in 21 Days," or "Supersize Your Chest," or some other inanity. There is no quick fix. To put on muscle mass requires hard work and determination.

If you were to actually read the article of building "Bigger Biceps," most likely there would be a list of exercises which would include barbell curl, concentration curl, alternating dumbbell curl, machine curl, and preacher curl all to be performed at three sets of eight to ten reps each. Of course, this would have to be in addition to all the other numerous exercises you're doing for all the other body parts.

Stop the madness. In this chapter, you will find the information to put together a routine that will pack on some serious muscle mass. Do not judge this program by the amounts of exercises, number of workouts, etc. or any other predetermined way. Keep an open mind. Less is more. If you use the right intensity, and I mean *heavy*, then these workouts work big time.

Lift heavy. Day in and day out. – **Pro Bodybuilder Ed Corney.**

Getting Ripped vs. Putting on Mass

The goal of any budding bodybuilder is, "I want to get huge and ripped." So many would-be bodybuilders try to achieve both at the same time with tons of aerobics and tons of lifting. The bodybuilder ends up over-trained and burnt out. First things first, train for mass *then* train for definition. The way you build a brick house is one brick at a time. So build for mass first, then cut your carbs and fats and perform some aerobic activity three times a week to get the definition later.

When training for mass, watch you aerobic activity. Try to keep the activity to low impact and low exertion - a little bike riding or some walking. If you do too much aerobic activity you hurt your chances to put on mass. Don't divide your body's resources between mass training and high impact aerobics.

Exercises

There is clear definition in Hardcore Natural Bodybuilding between which lifts are better for mass and which ones are better for shaping/toning. To get the most bang for your buck, you must use multi-joint or compound movements. Try to stay away from isolation movements, such as the lateral dumbbell raises, when trying to build muscle mass. Isolation and shaping exercises are out.

Listed in this chapter are the exercises best used for gaining solid muscle. The muscle groups are divided between the exercises that hit the muscle directly and the exercises that use the muscle as a secondary helper to aid in the lift. By understanding the exercises and how the muscles are affected, you will notice that even when the muscle is not a primary mover it can be hit with other lifts. You'll notice the biceps are getting worked during your back workout when you perform bent over rows and seated rows.

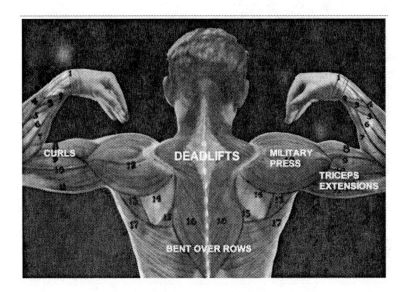

Biceps

> **Primary:** No substitute for the barbell curl with an EZ curl bar. Any dumbbell curl.
>
> **Secondary:** Any exercise involving a rowing motion for the back. Bent over rows, etc.

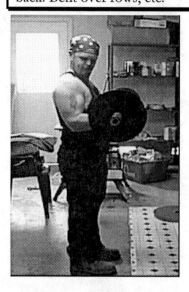

Exercise Spotlight: The EZ Barbell Curl

The Intro: The barbell curl with the EZ curl bar is by far the greatest mass builder for the biceps when performed correctly. A secondary stress is put upon the traps.

Finer Points: Grab the bar with a load that you can do for 6-8 reps and hold across your upper legs while standing. Keep your back straight, explode upwards until the bar comes all the way close to your chin. Hold for a second or two feeling the pump and let down the bar with control. Repeat.

No No's: Form, form, form. This exercise requires strict form. If you can curl 90 pounds with good form, but then curl 100 pounds with bad form, you are really still just lifting 90 lbs. Also, do not swing the bar up to get past a sticking point. If you do that you will lose all benefit of the exercise. Watch your lift speed, jolting the bar up very quickly and letting the bar fall back with no real control lessens the shock to the muscle. This is because momentum plays such a large part in the lift when done quickly.

Advanced Techniques: Cheat! What the hell are you saying? You just said not to cheat! When you get to 120 pounds-plus loads you may start to plateau. One way to get past a plateau is to use the cheating technique. When performed correctly, it works. On your last reps of your last sets when the bar gets to that 3/4 way up it hits that sticking point, then it is okay to arch a little to get the bar past that point. This is an advanced technique for the last reps not a correct way to do curls. Also try supersetting with dumbbell curls.

Triceps

Primary: Narrow grip machine pressdown. Lying triceps extension. French press. Narrow grip bench press.
Secondary: Any exercise for the shoulders or chest that requires a press, e.g. Bench press, Military press, etc.

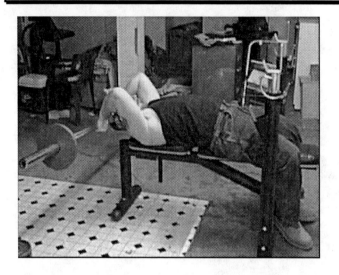

Exercise Spotlight: Lying Triceps Extension

The Intro: Performed with a barbell or EZ-curl bar. Puts stress on the entire triceps head. Great mass builder.

Finer Points: When performing the exercise, all you need is the bar, heavy plates, and a bench. While lying on a bench (with your legs at the end where your head is normally for the bench press), the barbell should be resting on your chest. Your head should be at the very edge of the bench. Grasp the barbell at six to ten inches apart. Push up and lower the barbell slightly past your head by bending your elbows. Don't let the weight travel far below your head - stop at a few inches past your head. Your elbows should be pointed at the ceiling. Push the weight back up to the starting position with little movement at your elbows. Repeat.

No No's: Don't let the weight drop quickly behind your head. Have control through the whole movement. Also don't let the weight go too far past your head, your elbows must point at the ceiling.

Advanced Techniques: Try straight barbells and EZ curl bars for different variations. Try different grip widths.

Trapezius

Primary: Upright row. Deadlift.
Secondary: Any exercise that pulls the shoulders downward while standing upright. Ex.) Heavy barbell curl.

Exercise Spotlight: Deadlift

The Intro: Great heavy hitter for the whole body. It's often called the upper body squat.

Finer Points: After thoroughly warming up, grab a barbell with an adequate load with your hands placed with one palm away from you and the other facing you. Bend your knees so they are over the bar slightly. Keep your back straight. Start the lift by driving your legs up. When you are standing fully erect, put your chest out and shoulders back. Bring the weight down slowly by bending your knees. Repeat.

No No's: For God's sake, don't start the movement by curving your back or bending over the barbell! You will risk a big time injury!

Advanced Techniques: Keeping the deadlift in your bodybuilding repertoire will help your other back lifts like the bent over row or the T-bar row.

Shoulders (incl. deltoids)

Primary: Dumbbell press. Military press. Behind the neck press. Any machine presses for the shoulder, preferably Hammer Strength®.
Secondary: Just about every exercise puts secondary stress on the shoulders.

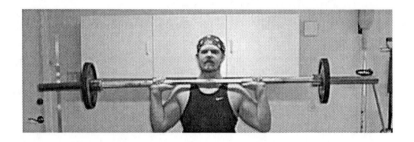

Exercise Spotlight: The Military Press
The Intro: Performed with a barbell and puts stress on the whole shoulder girdle. A great strength and mass builder for the shoulders.
Finer Points: This is definitely a heavy movement that requires warm up and pyramiding of your loads. It's best to use a rack that holds the weight at shoulder height. Once you've warmed up and are ready for heavier loads, take the bar off the rack. I find it's best to keep my eyes on a spot on the wall above my head and focus on it while lifting to help keep my balance. You can give the barbell a little help by pushing with your legs on the first rep to get it up. Then bring the weight back down and then

immediately push it back up. This helps you get into a rhythm. This is definitely a rhythm movement. If you pause too long on your shoulders on the downward movement with a heavy load it will be almost impossible to get back up on later reps. Repeat.

No No's: Do not use your legs to help get the bar up on any rep except the first. Also don't arch your back backwards. A little arching, and I mean very little, is okay. If you arch too much it takes the stress off your shoulders and starts moving some of the stress to the upper chest. Not only is this no benefit to the shoulders, it can be downright dangerous if you lose your balance.

Advanced Techniques: With a lesser load try pushing the weight up in front and bringing it down behind your neck. Push it back up again bringing the bar to the starting position. Alternating between a behind-the-neck-press and strict military press can be beneficial.

Chest

Primary: All grips for bench press. Hammer machine bench press. Dumbbell press. Dips.
Secondary: Military press.

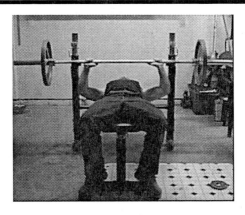

Exercise Spotlight: Bench Press

The Intro: The bench press is the granddaddy of all movements. Used by weightlifters all around the world to judge strength, it's a cornerstone of any of the hardcore routines. There's no substitute for the bench when hitting the upper body for mass.

Finer Points: Pull the weight off the rack and hold it above your chest with shoulder width grip. Take a deep breath and lower the bar slowly with maximum control. After the bar touches your chest, explode upwards (not too fast) while exhaling. Repeat.

No No's: Don't bounce the bar off your chest, arch your back, or lower the bar uncontrolled. Also on the last rep it's okay to let a spotter help you get past a sticking point but don't use a spotter on all reps, if you do that it means you just can't handle that weight. Of course, if you're stuck then a spotter can grab it.

Advanced Techniques: Vary your grip widths to hit different areas of the chest. Pyramid your loads. Try supersetting with dumbbell presses.

Abs

Guess what. Everyone in the world has the "AB six pack". It's just a matter of lowering your body fat so they can be seen. You can do crunches 3 times a week (try to do between 100-200 reps, four sets of 25,etc.) and see results. Just watch your diet. Try some weighted exercises.

Back

> **Primary:** T bar row. Dumbbell row. Lat pulldowns. Cable row. Bent over row.
>
> **Secondary:** Bench presses.

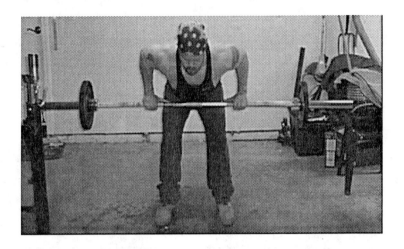

Exercise Spotlight: Bent Over Row

The Intro: Performed with a barbell and puts stress on the whole back. A great strength and mass builder for the shoulders, lats, and lower back.

Finer Points: This is definitely a heavy movement that requires warm up and pyramiding of your loads. When performing the exercise, the barbell should be resting on the floor before you begin the movement. Try lifting in front on a mirror so you can watch your technique so you don't get sloppy. Bend over and put your hands on the bar at shoulder width or a little wider than shoulder width. Bend your knees slightly. Keep your head up and looking forward. Lift the barbell to a point right below your chest and above your abs (the sternum area). Control the weight as it goes down, don't let it drop quickly or touch the floor. Repeat.

No No's: Your body will not be parallel to the floor during this movement., just very slightly upright. Don't round your back on the downward movement of the weight nor use lower back to jerk the weight upwards.

Advanced Techniques: When performing bent over rows, make sure that you always wearing a weight belt. Chalk or wrist wraps are helpful as well. When you get up to heavier loads, you can use your back a little, and I mean a *little*, to get the weight up.

Forearms

Primary: Wrist curls.
Secondary: Upright rows. Any exercise that requires you to grip.

Quads/Hamstrings

Primary: Squat. Leg press. Deadlift.
Secondary: Some amount of stress from exercises that require lifting while standing. Ex. Military press. minimal at best.

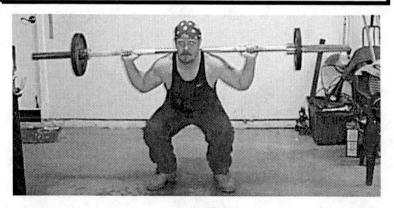

Exercise Spotlight: Squat

The Intro: Performed with a barbell. Puts stress on the entire lower half of the body. Great mass builder.

Finer Points: When performing the exercise, all you need is the bar, heavy plates, and a rack. Remove the bar from the rack by dipping your head under the bar and raising up. The bar should be resting across your shoulders. With your head and back straight, lower yourself to just below parallel, and push back up to the starting position. Repeat.

No No's: You must go below parallel when doing squats or you could hurt yourself later on. Also keep your head up and back straight to avoid injury. Remember to always warm up and have a spotter!

Advanced Techniques: A towel across your shoulders for the bar to rest on while lifting helps with discomfort with having the bar on your shoulders. Try different stances (wide or narrow) to work the inner quads and outer quads.

Calf

Primary: Calf raise
Secondary: Squat. Leg press.

Free Weights vs. Machines

I cater to free weights but you should use a combination of both. – **Pro Bodybuilder Ed Corney**

What!? I can have muscle gains and use machines? Yes. Proponents of free weights state that you cannot get quality muscle gains from anything other than free weights, which is untrue. These are the same people doing cable rows, lat pulldowns, etc. But I guess those are not machines, eh?

Your muscles react to intensity, which can come from many different stimuli. Your muscle doesn't care where the stimulus comes from, it just reacts. Put stress on the muscle and it will grow. *I'm not to saying free weights are not the best way,* just not the *only* way.

All machines are not created equal. In my opinion, Hammer Strength® machines are better because they move along the body's natural body lifting arcs.

Sets, Reps, Intervals

How many times have you seen people at the gym workout for one set and then spend five minutes talking bulls--t with someone else before lifting again? Serious lifters should be there with a business-like attitude.

When trying to put on muscle mass it is *very* important how much time is spent between sets with no more than two to three minutes rest at most. Hardcore Natural Bodybuilding is about sweating blood and pumping cold iron, not socializing.

For putting on mass, I suggest 4 sets of 6-8 reps.

- **First Set:** Warm Up. Light to Medium weight. If you have already warmed up on another exercise, there is no need to lift really light on subsequent warm ups for other exercises.
- **Second Set:** Pyramid load (adding weight to first set load) to get up to heavier weights.

➢ **Third and Fourth Sets:** These two sets are the majority of the work. These are your heaviest sets and will stimulate the most growth. The goal is six to eight reps. If you can achieve this, add weight to the sets until you have to work up to six to eight reps again.

Intensity

Ques: What's the biggest mistake that beginners make?
Answer: Trying to do too much with so many sets. Three hours is too long. After an hour you start tearing down the muscle. Just be consistent and don't give up too soon. – **Ed Corney.**

Intensity is the cornerstone of Hardcore Natural Bodybuilding. You must be focused and ready when you go to the gym. Lifting heavy workout after workout is tiresome. So your mind becomes the important deciding factor and will be the difference between success and failure.

How Heavy is Heavy?

As a Hardcore Natural, you lift the heaviest weight you can while still using good form. If you're benching 50 pounds more than your usual bench while bouncing the bar off your chest and arching your back, it's not going to help you achieve your goals. Maybe you can impress someone who doesn't know anything with your great feats of fake strength, but you're only hurting yourself. When you start cheating in your lifts, you're incorporating other muscles instead of the ones intended.

The load on the bar must be heavy for *you* not your buddy. As long as the last two sets are a struggle for six to eight reps then that's the goal. Often we compare ourselves to others, especially on how much we can bench press. Your bench press will get heavier but you must use good form on the loads you can handle. We throw around how much we lift like it's just a number. You might think, "I can only bench 180 right now". So what? Think of it like this: imagine your friend was moving and he asked you to pick up a box, a 180 lb. box. You would think, "forget it". It's not just a number. Just realize where you are now is not where you will be.

Program

The foundation of the Hardcore Natural program is the concept of less is more. Hit the body with heavy basic movements and then rest. The program is intense which will require rest. Working out three times a week is the maximum amount of time you need to be in the gym. Anymore than that and you're hurting yourself more than you're helping. The body needs rest. Smack the muscles with big lifts then let the body heal and grow.

The best mass exercises are multi-joint, basic compound movements. These lifts will edge your body towards growth more than any others. The Hardcore Natural formula is set up to hit the large muscle groups twice a workout and the smaller groups once a workout.

"But what if I only work out biceps once a week, will they still grow?" Yes, remember that the biceps are being used in your back exercises and possibly your shoulders as they are in upright rows.

Below are templates for you to create your own workout. You can substitute any exercise from the body part options. If the exercise is already written in the template, then you cannot substitute this exercise because it is one of the cornerstones to your growth.

Let's get started!

Basic Workout

Monday	Wednesday	Friday
Bench Press	Bent Over Row	Deadlift
Chest*	Back*	Shoulder*
Leg Press	Squat	Shoulder*
Biceps*	Triceps*	Upright Row
Dips	AB Work	AB Work

* Choose an exercise from **Body Part Option List**

<u>Note</u>: On Monday and Wednesday, you will notice there is a leg exercise halfway through the workout. The reason is it gives a break halfway through the workout for the upper body while still hitting the lower body. You will be refreshed for the last two exercises after the leg exercise.

If You Plateau On One to Two Exercises For Basic Workout

Stick with this workout as long as you can or until you plateau. We will define a plateau as an exercise you are unable to increase in weight. No matter how much you try you can't get six to eight reps. If this continues for four to five weeks, you could be plateauing. If this happens for just one exercise, try an advanced technique described later in the chapter. You may also want to check your diet to ensure you're eating correctly and getting enough rest.

If You Plateau On Three or More Exercises for Basic Workout

Take a week off and then try working out only twice a week with the Plateau Buster. Try this workout until you start plateauing once again. Then take another week off and go back to the Basic Workout at 75% of what you were lifting before you stopped and went to the Plateau Buster. Steadily increase your loads over your workouts to get back to where you were. Think of it as getting a running start to jump a large hurdle.

Plateau Buster

Monday	Thursday
Bench Press	Bent Over Row
Chest*	Back*
Leg Press	Squat
Biceps*	Shoulder*
Triceps*	Shoulder*

* Choose an exercise from **Body Part Option List**
Note: Many have tried the two-day-a-week workout without trying Basic Workout and made great gains.

Body Part Option List

Chest	Back	Shoulder	Biceps	Triceps
Incline Bench	Lat Pull Down	Military Press	EZ Bar Curl	Lying Extensions
DB Bench	Seated Row	Behind Neck Press	Alt. DB Curl	Machine Pressdown
DB Incline	T-Bar Row	DB Press	Preacher Curl	French Press
Machine Bench Press	One Arm DB Row	Machine Shoulder Press	Straight Bar Curl	Narrow Grip Bench Press

DB = Dumbbell

Plateau (Advanced Techniques)

You can't get past a certain load on a certain exercise no matter what? Sound familiar? When you've been lifting for awhile, you might start hitting a wall in your training. It's called a plateau. Plateaus are when your training has stopped producing gains. Your workout seems stale, tiring. Well, most of the gains you will make are in the first two years of your training. After that, gains are hard fought.

Here are some techniques that you can use to spice up that training to break that plateau.

Technique:

- **Rest** - This is one of the most underrated techniques of pushing past you limit. Have you been lifting a long time with no layoffs? Try taking two weeks off and come back stronger.
- **Check your diet** - Could what you're eating be holding you back?
- **Strength training** - High number of sets (5-6) with low reps (2-3).
- **Change the order of your exercises or the days** - A mental thing and it works.
- **Change of scenery** - Workout somewhere else.
- **Supersets** - Two exercises done back to back with little rest. Usually done between antagonistic muscle groups. One of my favorites.
- **Cut down rest between sets** – This gives you added intensity. Try it for awhile then go back to the normal time of rest between sets.

Adding muscle mass or breaking a plateau could be as easy as adding intensity to your workout. Intensity comes in many forms. You can use one of the above techniques or a combination: superset your exercises, add more reps, add more sets, or try strength training for a few weeks (less reps but more sets at a higher weight).

End

Arnold once said in one of his books, *Education of a Bodybuilder*, when lifting he would look at the bar and think: "You son of a b*tch, I'm gonna rip you off my chest, I'm gonna throw you over my head, I don't care how much you weigh. I'm the man who's gonna take you out."

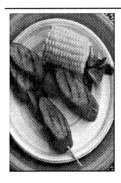

Chapter 6
Eat Meat: A Real Guide to Nutrition

If you read any popular bodybuilding magazine rag today they'll talk about diets that consist of 5,000 calories a day for mass? Yeah, right.

If you eat 4,000-5,000 calories a day you'll get mass all right - fat mass. Bodybuilders often tell you in the magazines their workout schedule, what exercises they use, and how they eat. They just don't tell you what drugs they're taking as part of their routine. Steroid growth requires lots of calories to undergo such a transformation, especially a lot of protein. If you eat 4,000 – 5,000 calories, they'll have to roll you out of the gym. Being a Hardcore Natural requires knowledge of a healthy diet for your training.

One of the keystones to any training is diet. What you eat can be one of the most overlooked parts of putting on muscle mass. Often budding bodybuilders think it's supplements that are going to get them to the Promised Land. Supplements are just that, supplements. If you do use supplements, use them as an additional *supplement* to a healthy diet.

Below is a diet that has worked for me as described by Adam Barlow, ISSA Certified Fitness Trainer.

The 40-30-30 Training Diet

The 40-30-30 diet consists of 40 percent of your calories from carbohydrate, 30 percent of your calories from protein, and 30 percent of your calories from fat. I will take you through a sample calculation so that you can compute your own daily requirements.

<u>Note for calories:</u>
- 1 gram of carbohydrate = 4 calories
- 1 gram of protein = 4 calories
- 1 gram fat = 8 to 9 calories.

If you are looking to decrease body fat, there are a couple of things to keep in mind.

- Set your final body fat percentage at an ideal level. Six percent bodyfat is bodybuilding competition level and the average weight-lifting buff is not going to reach this level - ever. Maybe somewhere between 10-12% is a practical goal, but one that will take a lot of diligence and hard work to achieve.
- The most effective way to lose bodyfat without losing lean tissue (very important), or to lose bodyfat and gain lean tissue, is to zig-zag your diet. Keep in mind that bigger muscles burn more calories than little muscles.

Let's assume you want to gain lean mass. I'll show you how to determine a proper diet and caloric content, but you need to calculate a few pieces of information:

A) **Lean Body Weight (LBW):** To determine your LBW, check out this site:
www.self.com/c_tools/calculators4/01home/calculators.htm
For our example here, I'll use 150 pounds LBW.

B) **Daily Protein Requirement:** Using a factor of 0.8 (three to four days a week weight training), I multiply the 150 pounds by 0.8 which equals 120 grams per day. This should make-up 30% of your total daily caloric intake.

C) **Total Daily Caloric Intake**: Stay with me here: 120 grams protein = 480 (120x4) = 30% of 1,600 calories. (40% Carb=640 calories or 160 grams; 30% Fat=480 calories or 53 grams).

D) **Meal Size and Frequency**: Divide the 1,600 calories over five meals to determine a basic meal size, but keep the 40-30-30 balance for each meal. According to my example here, a meal size will be: 30 grams protein, 40 grams carbohydrate, and 10 grams fat. Your meals should be consumed no less than every three hours. If you are going to sit on your butt for the next three hours after you eat your meal, eat less. If you're going to exercise within the next three hours, eat more.

E) **Zig-Zag for Mass**: Zigzagging is the process of modifying your daily caloric content based on your fitness goal. To continue with my example of gaining lean muscle mass, at a daily requirement of 1,600 calories, the weekly requirement is 11,200 calories. An "up-zig" day is a day when caloric intake *exceeds* the 1,600-calorie requirement. A "down-zag" day is a day when your caloric intake is less than the 1,600-calorie requirement. To gain the lean muscle mass without the fat, you need to have four to five "up-zig" days each week, and two to three "down-zag" days each week.

- **Up–Zig Caloric Calculation**: On the up-zig days, you need to add two calories per pound of LBW. My example here requires an extra 300 calories per up-zig day (150x2). Therefore, an up-zig day will consist of approximately 1,900 calories spread out over five meals. Or, you can keep the regular meal size and add a sixth meal consisting of 300 calories. The up-zig days should be eaten on the days when you train. You will provide your body with extra fuel for your workout and for the growth and recovery process.
- **Down-Zag Caloric Calculation**: On the down-zag days, you need to subtract two calories per pound of LBW. My example here requires eating 300 calories less per down-zag day (150x2). Therefore, a down-zag day will consist of approximately 1,300 calories spread out over five meals. Compute the 40-30-30 breakdown again using 1,300 calories. The down-zag days should be eaten on the days when you do not workout. Since you do not need the extra calories, this will help you body regulate and suspend fat accumulation.

F) **Monthly Adjustment**: At the end of a month, compute your LBW and then adjust your protein and caloric requirements accordingly. By the way, if you wish to lose fat, use the same methodology and calculations, but use two to three up-zig days and four to five down-zag days.

40-30-30 dieting is the best way to eat to burn fat and retain lean tissue. I highly recommend this as I have found that no other eating plan will produce the muscle gains or the fat loss that people are looking for.

Helpful Facts and Hints

Fact: The more muscle you have the more calories are needed to sustain the muscles.
Hint: Lose weight slowly, it betters your odds of keeping it off.
Hint: Take a multivitamin, like Theragran-M.
Hint: Eat fresh food, learn to count calories.
Hint: Don't miss breakfast!
Fact: Milk is a great supplement (2% milk, it is naturally 40-30-30 balanced).
Hint: Break up your meals into five small ones instead of three big ones. Prepare your meals ahead of time and use Tupperware® to store your portions.
Hint: Chopped lunchmeat from the grocery store made for pitas can be a great snack. Less carbs, more protein.

Truth on Water

Truth: Water is the most overlooked resource for the body. Lack of water can result in loss of muscle size since water makes up 72% of the muscle weight.
Truth: For glycogen (carbs stored in the muscle for energy), water is needed. For every gram of glycogen, 2.7 grams of water is needed.

Truth on Carbohydrates

Truth: Carbs are the primary source for muscle energy and the fuel for muscle contraction. There are two types of carbohydrates, simple and complex. Simple means that the body uses the energy quickly and complex is used when the body needs it.

Truth: A lack of carbs can result in the body using needed protein for energy. Too little carbs can make the muscles shrink as they lose glycogen. Too little carbs can hinder the body's ability to break down fat.

Truth: Eat enough carbs and drink plenty of water and save your money on Creatine.

Sources of Carbs: vegetables, beans, salads, fruits, whole wheat bread, rye bread, baked potatoes, slow-cooked rice, raw almonds, and nuts.

Truth on Protein

Truth: Many bodybuilders say, "Hey, you must eat 1.5 to 2 grams of protein per pound of bodyweight in order to gain mass". Untrue. Many medical studies have shown that 1 gram of protein per 2.2 lbs. of bodyweight is sufficient. Wow! I wonder why someone would tell you to eats loads and loads of protein? It's like companies want you to buy boatloads of the stuff, eh? Odd. It makes you wonder if there's some profit motive behind that?!

Truth: Proteins actually come in two different forms, complete and incomplete. Complete means the protein has all the needed amino acids that the muscles require. This means when something says it contains 12 grams of protein it doesn't mean your body can use all 12 grams. Some protein is better than others. Eggs have the greatest percentage of complete protein.

Truth: Protein does have calories! If you eat too much, it can be turned to fat. Diets too high in protein can result in a strain on the kidneys and liver, cause your body to lose calcium, and make you fat.

Truth: The body can only absorb 25-30 grams of protein per meal.

Recipes

Here are some my favorite recipes submitted to the website by readers.

- "My favorite source of protein is tuna fish. A 6 oz. can has 26 grams of protein, 0 carbs, and 1 gram of fat (Wieder can't beat that, or the price) as well as a large helping of vitamin B-6 (16% DV) and B-12 (40% DV)". (submitted by Nathan M)

- "Mix one can of tuna with 3/4 to a cup of nonfat cottage cheese together. Then mix one or two spoonfuls of salsa and a teaspoon of pickle relish together. You can mix all together or use the salsa and relish as a topping. It may sound nasty but actually tastes damn good. At 30-35 grams of protein with no fat, you can't beat it!" (submitted by gee1)

- "Cheap healthy and tastes good -- eat with oatmeal or whole wheat toast if you're not a zoner.

- 3 egg whites
- some chopped onion
- some chopped green or red peppers (optional)
- some broccoli (about 1 1/2 cups)
- 1 tsp olive oil

Sauté the onion and peppers for about 3 minutes in a frying pan, then add the broccoli and sauté another minute or so. Add a dash of water and put the lid on the pan and steam the veggies until the broccoli turns bright green. Take off the lid and let the water steam off. Add the eggs and stir 'em around just like you're making scrambled eggs. Total time's about 5 minutes if you're a quick vegetable chopper. Tastes great with a little Tabasco or fresh salsa.

Use organic vegetables, good quality olive oil and it's even better. Mushrooms, zucchini, cilantro all work, too." (submitted by Steve)

> "I've found that I get a good post body part pump when I eat eggs before I go to bed and have my nightly growth hormone release.
- 4 large Egg whites(raw)
- 8oz of Skim Milk
- 1 generous squirt of chocolate syrup

Mix together with whisk or blender (if you use a blender choose low setting). Pour into glass and drink. With this combination you get: 30 grams of protein, vitamin A&D, and low carbs from milk sugars and syrup

This is a better shake than anything you can buy in the store and as an added bonus it's real cheap. I'm talking $.70 a serving." (submitted by Graham L.)

➤ "Chop up some potatoes left over from dinner or whatever, scramble them with 1 yolk and 5 egg whites, then stuff it into a nice whole-wheat roll. 20 grams of protein from the egg whites + 3 grams from the yolk + 9 from the roll = 32 grams protein in only about 365 calories. I use the wheat roll because it's filling." (submitted by Keith P)

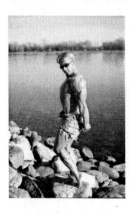

Chapter 7
So You Want to Compete?

Many gymrats have the fantasy of actually competing in a real bodybuilding contest but have no idea what it's really like. Read from Cabel McEdelberry's own words of what it's like to be a champion in the Natural Bodybuilding World.

From Cabel:

What's it like to be a competitive bodybuilder? It is the most intense physical and mental battle you could ever face. Without a doubt, prepare to set foot in a world that no one understands, support is unknown except from those that have made the journey. What is competing all about, well it's more than those few minutes you spend on that stage, let me try to explain....

Part I – The Journey Begins

"Build it and they will come!"

Profound words, but first before we don our posing suits let's think about the time it takes to sculpt a physique worthy of the stage. For me the time was two years. Was I ready? No, definitely not. The time it takes to build a body differs for everyone, but if you want to have a shot at a title you better do your homework. Go to some local contests, view the competitors, and try to talk to them off the stage. Somehow you need to objectively compare yourself to the competitors you have seen. How do you compare to someone who is about 4% bodyfat, dehydrated and has a better tan than you have ever had? Good question. When I figure this out, I'll never lose a show.

"You wanna get ready for a show? I think it would be easier to quit smoking!"

Contest dieting is the most demanding thing you'll ever try to do. Ever wonder what it would be like to have two full-time jobs? Ever go days with almost no carbs just for fun? It's just the beginning!

There are as many ways to prepare for a contest as there are competitors, but I will give you some details as to what I have done. I am constantly evolving and adapting, trying to unlock the pieces of the body's puzzle. The body is by far the world's most perfect machine, it will, without fail, adapt to everything if given enough time. So be prepared to do some research, knowing how to achieve that contest winning physique is a true science.

Contest preparation starts at about 14 weeks out from the contest date, yep that's right, 3 ½ months of agony before your 20 whole minutes of glory, still interested? Here is a general recount of what happens….

Week 14

- Before pictures.
- Body Composition – this will be used to determine amount of fat loss needed then divided between the weeks. (i.e. 1-2 lbs. per week usually)
- Monitor food intake to establish an average level of caloric intake.
- Eliminate obvious junk foods.
- Add a few low intensity cardio sessions after workouts.

Week 13

- Begin to adjust nutritional ratios, this has changed for me each year. I plan to start at 30% Protein – 55% Carbs – 15% Fat.
- Add a couple more cardio sessions. Probably about 30 min 5 times per week now.
- Start using vitamins. I use Multi-vitamins, 50mg B-complex, 3000mg Vitamin C, and 1600 IU Vitamin E.

Ok, you have made the initial transition into dieting at this point, now the fun begins. According to desired weekly weight loss we begin adjusting calories accordingly.

Week 12-8

Start adding salt to everything! Yeah, I know that sounds weird doesn't it? Damn, I felt dumb afterwards because it was there all along and totally makes sense. Most people believe that sodium is the cause of water retention problems but truly it is just the opposite. Right now your thinking I'm an idiot, it's ok so bear with me. Sodium is one of the electrolytes in our body and if any of these is imbalance you will suffer cramping and the puffy watery look. Most people maintain low sodium diets so our body adjusts to this. How? Well, it creates a hormone called aldosterone that tells our body to hang onto sodium to maintain proper electrolyte balance. See where I am going now? This is very simplified but basically it's like this, if you have high aldosterone levels you will hold water under your skin. So if we dramatically increase our sodium intake for a duration of weeks we can convince our body to lower natural aldosterone levels. Just wait, you'll fit this together later if you haven't already.

- Body composition every 2nd week to insure we are not losing lean mass. Must keep careful eye on subscap measure (Back). If it starts to increase it may be a sign of decreasing metabolism from calorie restriction, this makes it almost impossible to burn fat.
- Increase cardio to 40 min twice per day, first time must be before breakfast.
- Adjust nutrient levels, over a couple week span I lower carbs to about 40% and protein up to 30-40% while the remainder is made up of EFA's, which are not especially filling.
- Be hungry 24/7 - At this point I often use ECA stack 3 times a day more to curb appetite then anything else.
- Start tanning.

I don't usually lose much weight but for those that do. We will readjust caloric intake 12-14 times lean body mass to equal daily caloric intake.

Week 7-4

At this point my mind starts messing with me, I think I look like crap and am sick of dieting. Trying not to cheat, all I can think about is my next meal, and oatmeal is like candy.

At the 7 week mark a decision needs to be made, is my progress satisfactory? Am I on target? It's hard to tell, you constantly guess what your gonna look like in 6 more weeks. (You want to be ready a week early.) I try to apply how much I have lost and at what rate, which will not stay the same in coming weeks, but it is all you have for a measure.

If I feel I'm on target then I will likely not change things much, but usually I am so full of paranoia that I never feel I look right so will make the following changes:

- May increase cardio a bit, but damn I hate cardio so I don't unless I have to. That would put me at about 2 hours a day, split into 2-3 sessions. How do you feel about making time to go to gym 3 times a day?
- I will change my nutritional regimen to something much more fun. Yeah, right. I start using a 3 day revolving nutritional program, still eating 5-6 meals daily but carbs will fluctuate.

Day 1 – 6 meals consisting mainly of protein and EFA's. The only carbs I get today will be 1 cup cooked oatmeal and 1 ½ cups worth of salad before bed. Ever hear of ketosis? Ketosis is the point at which your body switches to fat as primary energy source in an effort to survive. In order to hit ketosis blood sugar must drop very low (i.e. no carbs) You will not quite make it to ketosis on one day with no carbs, which may help spare muscle, but will likely give you some of the most severe cravings you have ever had. Doesn't sound like much now but I feel like I have a carbohydrate addiction in the likeness of that of a heroin addict. At times I had Oreo cookies stashed in corners. You become someone other than you. But persist you must, in an effort to achieve.

Day 2 – Only difference between day one and two is on day two I will have a small piece of fruit instead of oatmeal and 1-2 cups vegetables with each other meal. A little better than day 1 but damn, by this time I am so tired of vegetables.

Day 3 – Day 3 is pretty much the same as day 2 except that for my last meal in the evening I will have a carb up meal. This will consist of oatmeal, yams, a banana, and yes more vegetables. The idea here, like training, is constant change. But constantly changing the level of carbs in your diet we try to get the body to continually try to adapt to what we are doing. In the process you burn a ton of fat!

Week 4-1

At this point I again try to assess my condition, you should be really lean at this point, nice and tight, very thin skin. Now I will change my diet slightly again to prepare for the carb depletion/load regimen in the last week. Somewhere in week 4 or 3. I'll bring my carbs back up to about 50% of total caloric intake. This amount then gets split down the middle, half starch, half-fibrous. Incorporating starches again at this point just gives the body a chance to adjust to using them again. This will insure the carb up process works well. Remember your body is about simplicity and balance so the more natural you can make things seem the better things will work. Natural, yet always changing, shocking the system. Confused yet?

My fat intake is somewhere in the neighborhood of 15-20% and is totally from EFA's (Udo's oil, Flax, CLA).

Protein intake is pretty much the same, about 30% and comprised of whole proteins.

Water should have been high through whole diet but now we crank it up even more, as much as you can drink. Usually try to get 2-plus gallons a day. You spend a lot of time in the can.

No more leg training at 14 days out.

These last weeks are where most competitors lose it, it's so close yet so far. Your body is very lean and it doesn't like it. Cravings are nuts and moodiness is common. Be prepared to hate your girlfriend/wife, your family won't like you and everything will *piss you off!*

Final Week

Here it is: the days that make or break you.
- Sunday at noon you will cut carbs to about 100g for the day total. This will still be half starch and half-fibrous.
- Monday you will cut carbs even lower, down to 50g for the day. It's not much fun, especially since you will be doing full cardio today and if you're a real man you'll even train. Nothing crazy, about 45 minutes of circuit training or so.

Remember all that salt you're eating? Well today you also cut sodium as low as you can.
- Tuesday is the same as Monday, but this will be your last day of training and cardio. From here it's time to coast.
- Wednesday is the fun day! Time to start the carbs. Today protein is something you eat if you feel like it, other than that it's starches every hour or so. I use yams, they are so sweet at this point.
- Thursday you should feel good, with lot's of energy, muscles feeling full. If you don't feel good, eat some more carbs. Otherwise it's just a regular dieting day. Today we'll cut water by about 1/3. 70 ml Glycerol with 16oz water twice today.
- Friday you should be ready, just make any adjustments necessary to ensure weigh-ins run smooth and cut water completely late afternoon. 70 ml Glycerol with 16oz water twice today.

Part II − The Time is Near, The Eve before Destruction

It's Friday night before the show, this is where the psychological battle begins. Tonight is the weigh-in. The weigh-in is the first time you see any of the competitors, you all gather in a warm little room usually at the host hotel. As you look around many thin tanned faces stare back, some peoples cheeks really cave in, this always psyches me out. As you peer around, the real test is to see if you can pick out the guys in your class. Soon the judges will call for each class to assemble behind a screen; soon it will be your turn.

When the time comes, everyone tries to be at the back of the line. To weigh-in you sometimes have to strip down in front of all the competitors in your class. Here you have your first glimpse of your competition, and they of you! It can get even worse if you are near the weight limit for your class and are worried about spilling over, if you weigh-in too heavy you have 30 min to try to make your class again. Ever sit in a sauna dehydrated? The weigh-in can leave you shattered or extra confident, I often end up somewhere in the middle. Nothing left now but to wait…

Judgement Day

The morning of the show finally comes. I'd like to say you wake early but chances are you didn't sleep the night before. If you're like me once you begin the dehydration process you have a constant headache and can't sleep. At about 4 AM I am so pissed that I can't sleep I usually go for a walk or practice my posing routine, thinking about the day to come.

When the sun finally breaks the horizon it is time to make the final preparations. I begin by having a decent size meal. It feels good to eat a bit more than you have been but I only drink as much water as it takes to get it down, a couple swallows at best. Soon I find myself standing in the bathtub again having my tan touched up with another coat of dye. Last but not least will put a little dye on my face.

The minutes pass slow as you wait to head to the theatre for the pre-judging. Waiting, thinking, resting…

Once you reach the theater you find your way to the dressing room where you lie on the floor, feet in the air, with the other competitors. Most are friendly, it's all done at this point, either you did your homework or you didn't. Often we share our dieting horror stories. As stage time nears you will see a variety of hocus pocus, last minute tricks to get that winning edge, honey, red wine, candy a few minutes before, niacin, that sort of stuff.

The runner comes in, your class is called, and it's time to begin the pump up...

Pump time!

The pump up room is the transition place. A few weights in a little room, all conversation ceases, it's time to focus. Everyone has different thoughts on what to do to pump up. I basically just focus on my worst bodyparts and try to pump them full of as much blood as possible. Lifting, feeling that inner rhythm, transferring my energy to that place we all know. It's like when you're in the leg press with thighs screaming, knees trembling and all you can think of is, "Yah man, this feels good I want more!" When the assistant comes its time....

The world suddenly spins on by, all your thoughts and dreams of that moment as you step on stage suddenly well up and wash over you as reality sets in, it's about to happen. You're only moments before walking on stage. The assistants are spraying you with PAM, smoothing your oil and making sure it's just right, your heart beats faster, pounding in your head, it's time to perform....

In the morning at prejudging you will all head out on the stage together. The judges will call for the compulsories. As you hit your poses you try to get a glimpse of the guy beside you, how is he posing? You squeeze, hard, expel all your air, your body is tight, your face looks calm, now hold it. The judging can be nerve wrecking, pose after pose, you tire, your body aches. The lights are hot. Dehydrated, you still sweat and your tan usually starts to run. The judges will move you around and you're always trying to figure out where you are in the placing. Usually, if you are in the center that is a good sign. After the comparisons are done you will do your freepose for the audience and then it's back to waiting….

In the evening things are a bit different, there is not really any judging, you will start with the freepose. This is incredible feeling, the stage is yours! People cheer and roar in admiration of every great pose. You are king and your loyal subjects pay their respects. Soon after, they call out the top 5. If you get called you once again go through the compulsories, and then it's time…. POSE DOWN!! The music is cranked, it's man against man, head to head, war. There can be only one, the heat and excitement is incredible, the audience roars, energy is found, hitting pose after pose. The pose down is the moment we all live for, it's the war of wars!

Once the pose down is done the placings are announced, one by one starting at 5th. Each time a name is called your spine tingles hoping it's not yours as you wait to see who remains the unannounced king.

Will it be you?

Note: This chapter was a look into the life of a competitive bodybuilder and was not meant to be an example of a diet to be followed.

Fortress

by eebowof (Yahoo Club)

Muscle on metal
Lift to survive
Mountains of mass
Your goal and your drive
Piling layers
Of meat onto bone
Building a fortress
Of flesh turned to stone

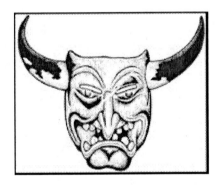

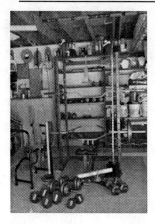

Chapter 8
Hardcore at Home and on the Road

When you're determined to get huge, you need a place to workout.

Home Gym

As a Hardcore Natural, you shouldn't care if you lift at the gym, in a garage, in a basement, at grandma's house, or even in the woods behind some tool shed. Being hardcore is in your heart and in your mind, so that goes with you wherever you go. So let's get started.

Memories, Memories

I remember when I got my first weight set when I was 13 or 14. It was a cheap narrow bench with those concrete Orbatron® vinyl weights. Orbatron, the lovely big brown round plates of concrete that were 7.7 or 14.2 pounds each. You had to become a big math wizard to calculate the loads. The bar was hollow.

Cheap crap, but it was lifting in my basement all by myself where I got hooked.

Later when I got a better set, I remember all the good times when my friends from high school and I would gather around and pump iron in my basement. We'd talk sports, girls, cars, girls, parties, music, and then back to girls again. We were there for one another and I think back to those times as some of the best.

When I was a bachelor and I had a roommate, all we did was party and chase women (we were older now, the "girls" were now women). Our life was all partying, nightclubs, women, and good times. But the one thing we had in our sparse bachelor pad was a weight set. We had it in the living room instead of a dining table. We would blast music and get serious with the iron. In my opinion, that's what it's really all about. Good times, being natural and hardcore, and lifting for the love of it.

Basic Needs

(Prices ($$) are based on prices found on the Internet)

- **Bench Press**: A must! Get one with wide forks, not the narrow ones where the forks are close to the sides of your head. One that adjusts for inclines is good. Accessories such as leg extensions and squat bars are up to you. ($$ = 150)
- **Olympic Weight Set:** These sets of weights with the large holes are better for balance and overall durability. This is the kind you see at the gym, you can purchase a 300-pound set including a barbell. ($$= 100 - 130)

Optional, but if you can get one:

- **Olympic Curl Bars:** Great for bicep curls and lying triceps extensions. ($$=35)
- **Dumbbells for Olympics Plates.** They're hard to find but great to have.
- **Power Rack**: I would put this in "basic needs" but it's a judgement call. If you plan to do heavy power-lifting movements like squats, then I strongly suggest you get one. ($$=200)
- **Plate Tree**: A great place to keep your weights when not in use. ($$=35)

The Other Essentials:

- **Rugs:** It's good to have a heavy-duty rug under your set. That way you don't crack the cement/floor or chip the weights.
- **Radio**: Pumpin' music is a *priority*! Nuff' said.
- **Portable Fan or Heater:** If you lift in the basement or garage, then the elements can be an issue.
- **Posters or mirror:** Adds to the atmosphere.

How To Save Money:

- **Brand Names**: Brand names mean crap! That means you can save money. The bench only needs to be sturdy and the weights only have to be heavy! Really, a 45-pound plate is a 45-pound plate is a 45-pound plate.

- **Cut A Deal:** You can find some great deals at used sports equipment stores and in your local newspaper's classifieds section under exercise equipment. Don't forget yard sales and online auctions!
- **Safety:** One of the biggest drawbacks to lifting at home is safety. I strongly, and I mean *strongly*, suggest you find a buddy to workout with. If not, lift as safely as possible. Don't lift any load you're not sure about. Always have a backup plan. Think to yourself, "If I get stuck what will I do with the weight?" If you're in the bottom position of a squat and you get stuck, how would you deal with it? The answer is to have a backup plan. Have something to place the weights on or somewhere to drop the weights. The best answer is to have a partner.

Commercial Gym

- **Type of Equipment** - Very important! You should already have in your mind before you go in a gym what type of exercises you want to perform and see if they have the equipment. If you're going to do squats, look for squat cages.
- **Quantity of Equipment**- Stay away from the "one-two" bench clubs. Bench presses are the most commonly used piece of equipment. If I see a club with only one or two benches, forget it! Also some clubs have only one or two EZ Curl bars, so check that out too.
- **Space** - Look for how much space there is in the weight room. If the equipment is really crowded together it can make for a tight fit when it's busy.

- **Ventilation** - I've gone into gyms and started sweating just checking it out. There's nothing worse than a hot gym. When you're really working out intensely you could get too hot or get a headache from a lack of oxygen. An added bonus for a gym is one that has two story ceilings instead of eight to ten foot ceilings.
- **Hours** - Check the hours! Make sure they are open to you any time you want to work out.
- **Price** - Pay for what you want to do. If you're not going to do Tae-Bo®, PACE®, Spinning, or swim in the pool, then *don't pay for it!* If all you want is a weight room, then pay for only a weight room. There's lots of "hole in the wall gyms" out there.
- **Crowded?** - Go to the gym during the hours you want to work out before you sign up for anything. That way you can see how crowded the gym is during the times you want to work out.
- **Location** - The gym has to be easy for you to get to or you probably won't go.
- **Parking** – Parking can suck. Find out where you can park if it gets busy.

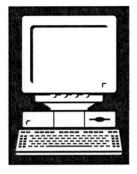

Chapter 9
Cream of the Crop: The Best Natural Bodybuilding Sites on the Internet

- ➢ **Adam's Natural Bodybuilding Page** – One of my good friends, Adam has lots of great personal info about his own training.
  www.geocities.com/Colsseum/Dugout/4143
- ➢ **All Pro Training** - Have a pro trainer make up a workout for you.
  www.allprotraining.com
- ➢ **Atozfitness.com** –Site has loads and loads of links.
  www.atozfitness.com.
- ➢ **The Brotherhood** –Home base for the Hardcore Natural.
  www.geocities.com/getoffmeyou
- ➢ **Classic Bodybuilders of the Golden Era**- See pictures of some of the old school bodybuilders before the advent of steroids.
  http://brianj1.tripod.com/classicbodybuilders.html.
- ➢ **Cyberpump** –. The authority on High Intensity Training (HIT). Has a "HIT Digest" sent via email.
  www.cyberpump.com

- **Fat Loss Secrets of All Natural Bodybuilders** - Great site on getting ripped.
  http://www.fatlosstips.com/.
- **Fig's Natural Weightlifting and Bodybuilding Page** - This hardcore cop from Florida has a great opinionated page on the sport.
  http://members.surfsouth.com/~figarola/index.html.
- **The Hardcore Brotherhood** – Best online forum anywhere.
  Clubs.yahoo.com/clubs/thehardcorebrotherhood
- **Hardgainer's Home Gym** – Great page for people who have a hard time putting on muscle.
  www.monmouth.com/~rclodfelter/hghghp2.htm
- **Henry Rollins** – Not a bodybuilding page but contains a great article written by musician Henry Rollins called "Iron and the Soul."
  www.geocities.com/SunsetStrip/Palms/4396/hrf.htm
- **Juslift.com** - A free web site which allows you to keep a virtual log of your weight lifting workouts. Also gives you charts, stats, etc. Can form a club.
  www.justlift.com
- **Muscleshock** – worth seeing for the graphics.
  www.webzone3.com/muscle/frame.htm
- **No Excuses** – A personal page with book reviews and some interesting and cool essays. Great reading.
  www.geocities.com/HotSprings/Spa/1779/NoExcuses.html
- **Thorax's Iron magazine** – Very Informative site. Been around a long time.
  www.ironmag.com

- **Truly Huge** – Forum, classifieds, and a weekly newsletter sent via email.
  www.trulyhuge.com
- **Wanna Be Big.Com** - Site has information of how to build a massive body while dispelling myths.
  http://www.wannabebig.com/

Prophet of Progress
by Bart Verheyen

No pain, no gain
When you think it's almost done you're just starting!
When you can't lift the weight anymore, push harder!
If you can lift the weight, if you can lift it to easy, take more!
Enjoy the pain : it's the prophet of progress

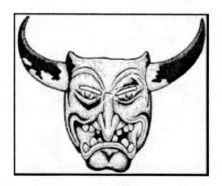

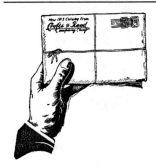

Chapter 10
Best Emails

Because of the nature of Hardcore Natural Bodybuilding, I often get emails from visitors to the site who are fed up with the commercialization of bodybuilding. The emails are full of emotion and frustration. Here are some of the best.

Email #1

Bros~ It's so good to finally find a site that isn't clogged with ads for some muscle in a bottle crap. I completely agree with your lifting philosophy. Only by lifting heavy and sweating will anyone ever grow quality mass. It's killer to finally know of a place that I can ask questions of someone that I know feels the same about lifting as I do. See you in the gym.

Email #2

The Brotherhood is FREAKIN' HARDCORE. At last a site with the same views that I have- eat healthy, get plenty of rest, and TRAIN HARD. 'ROIDS ARE FOR SISSY BOYS! My personal motto is Go Heavy or Sit on the Porch! If you ain't prepared to sweat blood then hit the stair stepper and if you want to get stronger, load the bar heavier! It ain't the size of the dog in the fight, it's the size of the fight in the dog! Heavy weights with low rep sets are where it's at, my Brother. And always remember the only thing that can defeat you is yourself. VAE VICTUS (Woe to the Conquered). Positive mental focus. I have had this mind set for twenty years. I just recently got on the net and almost soiled myself after checkin' out your site! I proudly uphold all the philosophies of The Brotherhood and would be honored to have my name placed on the Roll Call. As David Lee Roth says in one of the best iron pumping anthems ever:

> I got no taste for second place
> and I lead with my face, Yeah!
> I been places with my face
> ya wouldn't go without a pistol!
> I'm Relentless!
> Look Into My Eyes!
> Relentless!
> I Will Not Be Denied!

Keep up the awesome work. I'll be checking back often. THE BROTHERHOOD RULES!!!

Rock On, Brother...

Email #3

Ahhh, finally the sort of site I wanted to see on the internet; no more advertisements, no more "Please enter your credit card number to subscribe to our lame-ass publication blablabla", just the cold hard truth. I'm sick of seeing so much of what I love about bodybuilding being squashed beneath corporate strategies, marketing plans and sales figures, not to mention being made sick at the gym by the number of guys with Lat-syndrome (I've been looking for an appropriate phrase to describe these people. Thanks).

Email #4

Natural bodybuilding has seriously changed my life, my attitude and my motivation. Before I began I was a bit of an egomaniac with the martial arts and all, yet I had no motivation or self-confidence. After two years of weights, I've become humble, my motivation is through the roof and I have confidence in my self-achieved through goal setting.

I am ecstatic to see a hardcore, no bullsh-t website that offers free advice and inspiration. I've searched far and wide to find a web site that doesn't try and sell me anything or feed me a pack of lies. I too used to admire the 'big boys' in mags such a 'Muscle and Fitness'. I can't believe I wanted to look like those freaks. I have now come to the conclusion that bodybuilding, whilst invigorating to the mind, body and soul, is an art of illusion.

Email #5

My name is Mark. I have read your stuff, and I agree with everything. I've been bodybuilding for about 10 yrs. I am so sick and tired of all those guys at the gym, and at work, sticking a needle in their ass, and within three or four weeks, they pass you right by in strength, weight, and recuperation. Sometimes I feel overcome by all this, but then I take a look at myself, and say, "Everything I see in the mirror I worked for, and damn hard. All they have to show is ballooning muscles, pin cushion ass, and shrinking wallet not to mention what is in store for them in the future. I am so glad that I found you when I did. If there was a time in my life when I was teetering on the edge of roid-ville, it was just before I found your site. Now my values are reconfirmed. I am now a natural bodybuilder forever. Keep up the good work. Thanks, and I will pass your site to everyone I know. WEIDER SUCKS!

Email #6

I am finally glad to see a site that promotes the naturals as opposed to an unnatural freak. I went into the Navy in '91 at 150lbs and am now 180lbs. At first I wanted to get big fast and a buddy of mine that came in on a waiver for using steroids, who by the way played defense for UCLA, pleaded with me to take my time. He had to workout virtually everyday to keep his body from "sagging" as he called it. I took his advice due. Everyday I see huge guys with acne and receding hairlines in the gym and pity them. I am just glad that there is a site where honest healthy individuals can meet now and discuss real issues of natural bodybuilding. I thank you for this.

Email #7

I am an I.A.R.T. certified trainer, and an advocate of high intensity, but more than that I am a firm believer in reality. Most people are caught up in endless loops of useless routines that yield no progress, partially due to the fact that they are unwilling to swallow their pride, drop the weight back to a realistic amount, and use good form, partially due to the fact that they lack the determination to stick with something for more than a week.

Instead they will blame it on their genetics, their supplements, old football injuries, and my favorite, unbelievable time constraints that limit their training. But then again, if it wasn't for people like that, what would we do with all of the clever excuses that have been created over the years, and who would the supplement companies rape!

You can certainly hold your head up for taking a stance, we need more dedicated and realistic websites like this!

Rock On

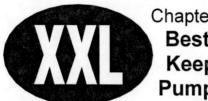

Chapter 11
Best Mantras to Keep the Blood Pumping

Often when the chips are down we look to a catch phrase to keep us motivated - a phrase that defines how we feel about a certain topic. Here is a collection of my favorites.

- If you're not getting better than you're getting worse.
- The journey of a thousand miles begins with one step.
- The only failure in life is the failure to TRY.
- Failure is not getting knocked down, failure is when you don't get back up.
- Pain is temporary. Pride is forever.
- He who endures, conquers.
- Strength through pride then pride through strength.
- May God have mercy upon the iron, because I won't.
- Limits are for people who have them.
- Don't do your best. Do what it takes.
- If you can accept losing, you can't win.
- The greatest happiness is to crush your enemies and drive them before you. To see his cities reduced to ashes. To see those that love him shrouded in tears. And gather to your bosom his wives and daughters. – Genghis Khan, 1226

The Hole
by tolkein_1999

As I fell asleep after a brutal training session, I had a dream. Kind of hazy but quickly came into sharp view. It was the perfect gym. I parked outside and walked up to a place called "The Hole". It looked like an abandoned warehouse. As I walked up to the gym, I could hear hardcore music pumpin' from the stereo, sounded like AC/DC's "TNT" but I'm not sure. There was no membership. All I had to be was Hardcore, a tribe member, and knowledge of the Creed. I was admitted past the Gatekeeper.

I went to the lockers. There were no lockers just piles of clothing on a bare cement floor. There were no need for lockers and security. After all, no one steals from their fellow brothers.

As I went into the gym, it was heaven. Hardcore tunes, no guys with lat syndrome, no spandex, no steppers or bikes, just heavy weights as far as the eyes could see and fellow members of the Brotherhood training heavy and helping one another. I never had to wait for anything. I never had a problem finding a spotter. We were all there for one another. We were hardcore. We were one. We were a Brotherhood.

This was more than a gym. It was Our House.

A Note from the Author

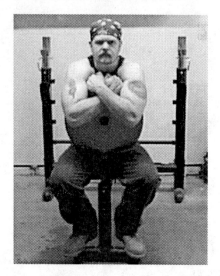

I hope you have enjoyed this book as much as I have enjoyed writing it. Remember that being a Hardcore Natural is in your heart and mind and goes with you everywhere. Go Heavy or Go Home.

Rock On!

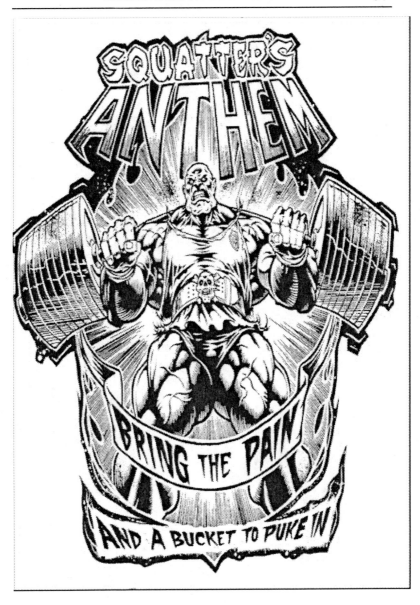

Courtesy of **Iron Asylum**. Visit **www.ironasylum.net** for more awesome designs!